LESSONS
FROM MY FATHER
FOR MY SON

A CAREGIVER HANDBOOK

CHRISTINE CARLISI MANZI

authorHOUSE

AuthorHouse™
1663 Liberty Drive
Bloomington, IN 47403
www.authorhouse.com
Phone: 833-262-8899

© 2024 Christine Carlisi Manzi. All rights reserved.

No part of this book may be reproduced, stored in a retrieval system, or transmitted by any means without the written permission of the author.

Published by AuthorHouse 11/27/2024

ISBN: 979-8-8230-2353-5 (sc)
ISBN: 979-8-8230-2352-8 (e)

Print information available on the last page.

Any people depicted in stock imagery provided by Getty Images are models,
and such images are being used for illustrative purposes only.
Certain stock imagery © Getty Images.

This book is printed on acid-free paper.

Because of the dynamic nature of the Internet, any web addresses or links contained in this book may have changed since publication and may no longer be valid. The views expressed in this work are solely those of the author and do not necessarily reflect the views of the publisher, and the publisher hereby disclaims any responsibility for them.

This book is dedicated to all the compassionate warriors who are taking care of the beautiful people they love

PREFACE

TIMELY REFLECTIONS

I have always been an observer of people and events. For as long as I can remember, I have noted my observations and reflections in journals. Much of the material in this book was excerpted from these journals. The journal entries were written at various junctures in my life. Therefore, the dates may seem confusing because they are not presented in chronological order. I chose to order them based on content, not when I wrote them. Each musing or poem is a message to my son.

> "I'm captured in the carousel of time." Joni Mitchell, "Circle Game"

> "Youth cannot know how age thinks and feels, but old men are guilty if they forget what it is to be young." Dumbledore

> "I know God will not give me more than I can handle. I just wish He didn't trust me so much." Mother Teresa

INTRODUCTION

My darling father fell out of his hospital bed in Florida, which resulted in a hematoma on his brain. After a long rehab stay, he returned to his Florida apartment in the care of private nurses. It soon became clear that he needed to come home to NY. He lived with me for a time and I learned lessons from that experience. Many of them I learned after the fact, upon reflection. When you are in the midst of caring for a parent who needs you, it is very hard to deal with the everyday challenges. To actually learn something at the same time is unlikely. Until you have been there and back again, you are really just flailing in the dark for most of the time. Even the most caring and concerned child can never fully understand what a parent needs. This is true, even when our parents are "young".

When the parent is the child and the child becomes the parent, things really get muddled. As I read through some of my reflections about my father that I wrote right after he died, I realized they can be quite dark. I had never thought about how I would operate in this situation and I feel as if, had I known more about aging or caring for the aged, I might have been better prepared. Maybe I would have had less regrets when all was said and done. I do not know. I do know that I tried my best and all of us have to take comfort if we have tried our best, in whatever we do. I do hope that as one reads about these lessons from my experience and the experience of others, it might at least enable them to think about the different roles we might play in life.

It is in this spirit of reflection that I want to share lessons I learned from my father as a possible guide or roadmap for my son and others as they navigate the possibility of having to be in the challenging world of caring for aging parents. I consider this handbook a gift from my father. That is not to say I did not also learn many lessons from my mother.

My mother died 10 years before my father when she was 74 years old and completely competent and independent. As a result, I never became the "parent" to my mother. However, watching my mother as she aged taught me many lessons, which were layered upon the lifetime of lessons she gifted me with every day. I consider what she taught me to be a treasure trove of information for any person who wants to truly love others, whatever their ages.

Parentless now for many years, I think of my mother and father every day, I thank them both for the lessons they taught me, and I pray for them every night.

REMEMBER I WILL DIE

You will be caught up in caring for me and your own family
You will forget
It will surprise you
I might "come through" some episodes
You will be fooled into thinking that's how it will be
You, dragged to a hospital in the middle of the night
Me, getting through the night and getting back home at some point
Silly really
Prepare for my death by treating me as though it is imminent
This approach actually works for every one we know
But truly, chronologically, we are closer every day
I might be melodramatic about my aches and pains
or I might be stoic and quiet
Either way, tell me sincerely that you are sorry that I do not feel well
And you wish you had a magic wand to wave over me and make me well
Then kiss me
And do not worry

2002

In my early fifties, I am at the age when I can try to imagine my future as an older person.

My father always said the fifties are your heyday…enjoy them

I can remember my mother, hobbling across the baseball field, bent but hurrying before the outfielders took their positions

Embarrassed and determined

Probably worrying about where the bathroom was located

Smiling nonetheless as she laid eyes on her beautiful grandson running out to left field.

2005

You would think that I'd have learned my lesson by age fifty six
There is no controlling destiny
Simple, yet the key to living a life to the fullest
Sure, go to the hospital Pop, I think it is a good idea-just to check your medicines-benign
We trust Dr. Ali to do his thing
He loves you after all
But no one can love you enough to cheat Fate
Or poor choices by hospital staff
To give you a "little bleeding on the brain"
To disturb your carefully guarded delicate universe
You knew, but you chose to trust and love anyway
Sacrificing your fragile hold
Jumping into the abyss
Now what?
I am SO SORRY Pop.

6/08

I understand better every day as I approach a new birthday, almost 60, what you need to know in the future. Even though it doesn't make a lot of sense to you, give me prune juice every other day. It truly will improve the quality of my life. Leave flushable wipes in the bathroom. Know that I am aware of and afraid of my failings, even if I stubbornly try to appear as if they don't matter. Soothe me in any way that you can imagine. Stop and listen, even when you do not want to. Repay me and your father for the time we gave you, even though you have forgotten most of those moments as they blended together into the fabric of who you have become.

Teach your unknowing children how to love an old person who is not a stranger to you, though the familiar ways in which you know us may be dimmed. Remember who we were when we were vibrant, but also remember who we became, even with all of our faults and failings, as we are one and the same. You will be frustrated and saddened by who we become, but try to accept us and your role in our lives. This is very hard to do because we are both afraid, but there is no controlling or changing it. I am no reflection of you or the person you once knew. I am only the best I can be. I think this is the true generation gap. Don't "miss me" because I am still here! Only your gentle touch and love will be the connection we have and I crave. This parent-stranger who needs you so.

WHATEVER

Long before my Dad needed my help, he started saying, "whatever"
When I think of it now, he was probably in his sixties at the time
We made a sweatshirt with "Whatever" emblazoned across the front in bold colors and laughingly presented it
We thought it was apathy, or worse, disregard for important things
Alternating "whatever" with "this too shall pass" seemed somehow irresponsible being uttered by a heretofore concerned-about-the world erudite man
But I find myself these days saying, "It really doesn't matter" quite often
Much to the chagrin of my detail-oriented older engineer husband
Who basically thinks I do not care enough about things.
Not that I was ever very detail oriented
As you age, maybe especially after you retire, the "important" things smelt down like a precious gold ring into a gleaming puddle
What is left is the memory and significance of that ring, not its monetary value

What is important and keeps my attention now are the beautiful basics

One can see them more clearly once the detritus of life washes away on the tide of time

We are very busy working, raising a family, "becoming"

For most of our lives

If we are lucky, it is in the whatever years when we can hear the quiet, ponder the natural world, excise the worries of the world that are all too consuming

Maybe focus on our own place in it

Connect with others in new ways

Treat ourselves to NOW

Knowing much about mortality as it hovers over us and our loved ones every day

Try to let go before it is too hard to think or to get around

BE in whatever capacity you are able

Say "whatever" when you can now

Don't wait until you are sixty or retired

Turn off the phone

Ignore some of the news blasts

Find new ways to enjoy life

New ways to handle stress and worry

Hug more

Be kind to yourself

Bolster yourself

You might not get to have whatever years

6/18

Ten years since Dad left

Taking with him lessons I could have learned

So intelligent, such a natural teacher always

As I leave my 60s, observations about how to care for an elder are coming to me through my personal failings and through my contemporaries' experiences

"Is your husband doing this?"

"I feel crankier than I have ever felt"

"Every day is a new ache or pain. You have to laugh!"

I know now that warm water feels so good as I let it run over my hands in the sink. Arthritis.

The new higher toilet is a Godsend.

It is getting very hard to open containers. It is a good thing that I have a thingamajig that helps me

I am thinking that soon I should buy shampoo that is also a conditioner since I can't read the labels in the shower without my glasses.

I remember when we visited Dad's apartment in Florida many years ago; he had only conditioner and was using it as shampoo. Luckily, he was graced with an amazing head of hair and it didn't seem to matter what he washed it with. I do not think that washing my hair with conditioner would go well.

I find that I am happy to use the handrail in the shower that we had installed for Dad when he lived with us.

7/19

I just recently celebrated my 70th birthday. A septuagenarian! Hard to grasp, really. A significant portion of my life is done; a wonderful life, full of love, joy, adventure, accomplishment. Dreams fulfilled.

My high school classmates and close friends are dying. The idea that we are on the last leg of this journey demands reflection. What do I do now? Contemporaries are getting stents and TIAs. Did I do enough? How do I live every day to the fullest? How will I navigate the fears and the losses?

8/08

Perhaps because I couldn't see the dying
Perhaps we never can, even when a person struggles every day
85, lost and missing his essential core
Or, down to 70 pounds
Gritting against the pain inflicted by our cancer cures
Embrace the signs
The inevitability, the urgency
To help you to remember
To love harder
Show it more clearly
Allow Death to strengthen you for the daily challenges of living
For those challenges are monstrous tasks to undertake
Find other folks to help you
Sometimes, if you are lucky, they will come forth from the past
Gentle Jonathan laughing and talking with Pop every day until we could hire a caretaker
Cousin Meggie lovingly shaping Pop's unruly hair
Careful to get it "just right" for him
Running her fingers and scissors through that beautiful silver hair, his pride and joy.
Touching, talking laughing
Not too many people will take the time to help you
Busy with their own lives
Their own aging parents

And when you feel the most desperate, try to know that if I wake up again tomorrow
You have at least one more chance to love me the best you can.
Remember that I always told you to try your best
Be gentle with yourself
When I am gone, you will talk to me in your dreams
You will miss my smile
You will see clearer, what you could have done while I was still here
Read these pages and consider them
I wish someone had taken the time to pen their understandings
Before I was thrust into the everydayness of the task
With hardly enough time to think
Never mind to consider how not to have regrets later on
When I got back the precious think-time again.

8/24/07 PART I

It is impossible to grasp this particular loss

Oh, Mommy, how did you manage it?

High notes an integral part of who you are

97% is not good enough

To keep you whole

We lose each piece every day

Of Who we are

And somehow we are made to go on

Get strong once again

I think of the boys who

Have no legs

Scarred beyond recognition

And the stories of their bravery and desire to live

To become one again

Without the lovely gait

Or the baby smooth forehead

Warriors us all in the battle to preserve our inner selves

Whoever they might be

Without their physical counterparts

That we have come to know and love

Despite their fleeting presence

The cancerous cells looming always

Threatening to take them away
And
Change
Forever.
The essence of our lives.

8/24/07 PART II

Or is it the essence

That remains constant

That core that thrives despite the losses

That seed of Being, buried deep, protected

Does the absence of familiar parts

Strengthen the Self

Allow it to shed vagaries

Move to a more substantial place

In our consideration of life and its meaning?

Survivors seem both fragile and permanent

In a way those without tribulations are not

They smile wryly at our worries

Wonder how we can be so shallow beading

Over inconsequential mundane concerns

Knowing.

8/24/07 PART III

Or are we ultimately only the sum of our parts
So, as age itself robs us of smooth skin
Replacing it with wrinkles and age spots
As our legs give way under us
And we cannot recall a word
Does the chipping start?
Ever so imperceptibly that we are taken unawares
Of the process
And thus left hopelessly helplessly unable to reconcile old age
And then, when we hear that our bodies are failing us
From the Doctor at Sloan
We are shocked and saddened by this turn of events?
Unable to grasp this obvious loss
We are vital and have only just begun
After all.

8/24/07 PART IV

Then look at the baby who fails to suck
"Failure to thrive"
And answer the questions we older adults ask
Who grew fat at our mothers' breasts
And ran through the poppies chasing butterflies
Read our books
Became who we are as we brought new life into the world
Grunting and rejoicing at the miracle of this child
Who thrived and provided us Pieces of self
We had never imagined
Child who would take our "whole" presence for granted
For he could not possibly understand yet
The chipping process
Child who one day will cry for our losses
While we sleepwalk through our days
Waiting to join those of us who have already gone
Looking for who we were when we held him in our smooth and spotless arms

8/24/07 PART V

Look around

Find the pieces of those who have picked up the pieces

Sewn together a meaningful life

When everything meaningful was taken away from them

Learn.

Listen.

7/01

Revel in your youth
Enjoy it, treasure it
But feel no superiority
Because of it
Youth is a gift, not something earned
That allows you to laud it over those who also had it long ago
Instead, take a minute to reflect on those of us who laugh
Despite the aching of our bodies
Persist when we look in the mirror
And remember, as though it was yesterday
What it was like to be you.
Ah youth
You invigorate
Touch my heart
With your outstretched arms
So pure and unknowing
Knowing travails that in the end
Are laughable insignificant
Against the black dawn of aging
Deteriorating
Wisdom that you too
Will wither and die
Lamenting

Laughing
Imploring
Learning about the strength of loved ones
Grateful
Learning more about stamina, will, patience
Despair and the depths of joy
Family
Myself.

2/98

I've noticed ever since my mother died
When I lay down to sleep
Mortality throbs in my ear
Pressed to the pillow
Echocardiograms
Swooshing beats, murky and thick
I can say my Hail Marys to that beat
Some nights it soothes me
Reassuring. I am alive
Other nights I want it to stop
Abruptly
With no warning
Closed eyes, open mouth
Lifeless, yet so ultimately life-like relaxed
I see her, finished with her pain
Beautiful.

7/01

He lays there wondering
Looking at the ceiling
And alternately closing his eyes
Hands clasped on either side of his neck
Thinking of Mom off the piano bench
So close to his head so far away
Listening with those musician ears
To the life beat within him
Feeling the pulse of the carotid pushing violently against his palms
Scared and surprised at the ferocity of his own life
Longing for the time when the beat went unnoticed
There but only to allow him to do what he wanted to do
Not
Invade his privacy
Intruder
Shouting its limited existence in his ear
Alone

7/02

I must be royalty

I see the blue blood in my veins

A map on my hand

Topographical really

Hills and dales

Bulging mountains

Bas Relief Rivers

Scratched ravines in a desert

Earth cracked, crackled

Smooth only where the prominent rapids flow

8/17

Tendons stretched
Attachments tentative
As you go about your day
Wondering
When you'll snap

MOM

That incision looks so painful
Yet you laugh with us so freely
Those of us who can laugh without pain
Taking for granted the uncut flesh
And lack of sutures

"MEMORIAL" DAY

Regrets, I have some…

Dad is gone

I wrote about my friend

Needing to celebrate

Each ravaged cough

And a few years later

I dragged an old man

From place to place

Tired and thinking too much

About the next day

As if it would come

Only to add to my burdens

And not to give me a chance

To bask in his smile

Or hug or kiss him every minute

Loving his tainted presence

For it was fleeting as is all

Of our time

In my heart of hearts

I didn't remember to love him enough

Going through the motions

Acting as if I were taking care

Providing for his daily needs

Instead of just loving him with all of my might

How could I have done both better?

6/30/07

I see him there

Peacefully sleeping in the sun

The warmth pouring over him

Dreaming.

I stroke his calm forehead

Murmuring

I should have stroked it more

While he was breathing on his own.

7/4/07

I see you through the lens
There together laughing easily
Caught in a moment of joy
Youthful, full of promise
I think of you in "Elsewhere"
Arm in arm
Eyes twinkling
At a luscious dinner table
Of course, big band music is playing
Friends and family are in the room
Celebrating your reunion
And toasting your love
All embracing the charming couple
Who were apart for too long.

9/2/07

HUG me a lot while you are taking me from doctor to doctor
Infringing on your precious and vital time
Away from your own family and obligations
Your dreams for yourself
Tell me you love me and stroke my forehead
In your job of caring for me
Listen to my repetitive stories with glee
For you won't hear my voice forever
The voice that sang to you when you were helpless
Cooed when I diapered you
Told you how much you were loved from the day you were conceived
Try to remember through the trials of my lack of remembering
Through my inability to hear you
See you
That you are whole in my heart and
So am I.
That I have loved you so
Be patient and kind even
When you want to scream and cry out
That you can't take it anymore!
The burden is too great
Too sad

Too frustrating
For I know today that you will be more content
More happy
When I am gone
If You Can Do These Things.
I know too late
From learning about my own patience and kindness
Through my loving father
Who I didn't love enough at the end
I know and I will pass it on, without shame.
No one had told me these things.
Should have just hugged him more
Rubbed his aching body
Washed his feet.
Like Jesus did.
I could have talked less to doctors and nursing homes and assisted living personnel
And tried to let go of what I thought was best for him
A crazy idea really
Could have deferred to his understandings of what he was, who he was, what he needed
Could have stopped lamenting his losses
Making faces when I didn't understand
Could have complained less
And celebrated more the fact

That he knew me and still looked directly into my eyes
With his bruised face
And told me he loved me.

7/09

If I say a crazy thing, like, "Gee, I'd love a cigarette!" don't look at me as though I am crazy. At my age, I should just be able to get one or a whole pack and smoke it, one by one, circles surrounding the tip as I exhale extravagantly. But I am no longer able to drive or walk to the Corner Store. Even if I could, I probably wouldn't remember how to get there or where my cash was. Make sure I always have a wallet with money in it and a pocketbook available even if I never get to use it. My whole life has existed inside the zippers and pouches of pocketbooks, devices that order a woman's universe, help her to mother…"I'll give you fifty dollars for a tweezers, one hundred for a band aid…" Let's make a deal! "Have you got a safety pin or a tissue?" While you are at it, if I am still mobile, make sure my pocketbook is not too heavy – gravity does enough to weigh me down.

6/18

You know that I do not know how to fix my computer
Watch a movie
Put captions on the TV while I am watching
Your father always did these things
I may not even be interested in these things at some point
Please make sure that I can access music as it has always been my lifeline. Right now, I do know how to command Google and Alexa to play music, but will I always?
Share hard copy pictures
They will most likely delight me and help me to see the past through the haze
Keep young people around me for I have drawn strength and joy from young people for my entire life
Real human interactions will always trump virtual for me
Flowers have always provided me with happiness and a reminder that life is good
If I am still cooking, organize my kitchen so that everything is easy to reach and as light weight as possible
Gone are my days of using heavy expensive pots and pans China plates and crystal
I'll be happy with paper plates and plastic glasses

6/18

I know I am a burden
I know you will soon be free of me
But I need for you to still love me like you did
When you skipped next to me, your little hand enclosed in mine so long ago
Me your hero and protector
Innocent and true, thankful that I was in your life
So, say I love you first
Try to really mean it
Because whether you know or not, I will.

2/08

I was so busy
Making lists, appointments, arrangements
To remember that smiling beautiful face
That shed its light on me for my whole life
Instead I saw the hooded eyes, the worried mouth, the confused brow, the sorry little boy.
I did not stop long enough to see the glimmer there when he ate something he loved, thought about the old neighborhood or his Aunt Lena
I could have looked harder to see the displaced person
Independence shredded piece by piece
Until I saw the reluctant eater at the institutional dinner table with institutional food and mock friends all in the same boat
His chopped Samson hair sticking up in clumps, mangled by an institutional barber.
Broken.

1995 MCDONALDS

Staring through the arches in the front window
Rubbing arthritic tender hand
So much care and coordination went into dressing
Obviously the habit of a once business woman
Children, families chatter happily
The Ancient slowly spreads the prepackaged butter
On an English muffin
And quietly
Feeble
Bites of mashed egg
Butter smeared on her chin

I AM YOU

You hobble along the country road
Pushing your walker over pebbles and fallen leaves
Your cataract eyes strain to read the fat and salt
contents in the cans in the aisle at the A&P
You talk on the phone
Your friend who is recovering from a bypass
And you worry about the wife's blood pressure
TV glaring.

Addendum
When a young person dies
We realize that we all so easily assume that we
will grow old
We worry about our gradual demise instead of
embracing the now,
Forgetting that we may never have the opportunity
to be that blue-haired woman.
A few days after happy, young, Holly is killed
While sitting on a park bench overlooking the Sound
I am struck by the fact that we so easily assume
Old age will be a part of our experience
Considering this I embrace fiercely
The Now
Lose the worry of my gradual demise
Look at the blue-haired woman
With a different eye

BORN OF YOU/DAD

Your blood running through my veins
Your genes imprinted
Your life impacts me to the core
The center that you talked about as if in a dream
Of tortured Japanese soldiers
Grimacing leaving a snapshot on your soul
Grunting and crying out
And yet I couldn't understand
Didn't sympathize enough
Drama king.

Dad would love to go out for lunch. He'd take 40 minutes to decide what to eat. And then, after a few bites, be finished. Do not be annoyed if I do the same thing. The social aspect of lunch or dinner "out" is the thing. Don't grill me your favorite steak. I will have trouble chewing it and I will know that I have hurt your feelings when I can't eat much of it. Learn how to make yummy soft foods when you cook for me.

1/07 MOM

I couldn't understand why the old piano bench, long forgotten in the back room, was surreptitiously moved into the guest room when Mom and Dad came to stay. Why do you need a chair or a bench in the bedroom? Boudoirs with lavish chaise lounges were a thing of the past, when people actually did more in the bedroom than fall exhausted into a bed after a too busy day. Perhaps chats and reading, one hundred brush strokes on long thick black hair, or crocheting.

Or, as I am discovering, among so many other things, a place to sit while you pull on your panties, which is easier than hopping on one foot while your knee pops out of place or your arthritic back strains reaching a toe into the leg hole. I suspect that as I grow wiser with age I will learn other uses for a bench in the bedroom and maybe know someday why my mother sat on that piano bench as she died, just before bedtime.

4/9/20 MOM

Her arthritis bends her in half and yet she moves as quickly as she ever did
Seeing to everyone's needs
Cooking favorite meals
Always with a smile
Always supportive
You might catch her once in a while with a melancholy look on her face
Or a wince from the pain
Because she thinks deeply about life and her journey through it
But always comes back to the sunshine, spreading joy.

4/3/14

Take me for a pedicure every two weeks
Send me Nana notes in the mail
Don't let my house fall into disrepair
Get someone to clean my windows
Make sure I don't wear clothes with stains on them
Caress my arm. Hug me
Smooth the frown from my face
Touch will keep me happy
If you have an animal, bring her to visit me
So I can pet and coo
Read to me
Make sure I have several pairs of glasses so I can always see
Tell me about what is happening in your life, your family, your work
Talk to me even if you are not sure that I can understand you
If I simply can't hear you, repeat what you are saying until I hear you correctly
These are huge requests because they not only take time, but they take forethought and planning
Surprise visits! But, maybe call first!

9/2/07

See to it that someone plucks my chin hairs

Does it lovingly

Because they are a part of me

Put there by God to keep us humble

To tell us we are all the same

But at different stops along the road

You are me and I was you

Even though you've yearned for chin hairs as a symbol of your manhood

From when you're a little boy

And I lost the ability to even see them in the magnified mirror to pull them out

Make sure my hair is combed

That I am clean

Don't tell me what to do

Open the blinds to let in the light

When I might want to ponder my mortality in the dark

I know that I know nothing of those numbered days

And neither will you until you reach them

Hope that the lessons your mother learned from her parents

Have touched you too

And been handed down in some way

To the children you have
Who will someday help you out of the tub
And hopefully smooth some lotion over your crepe skin
Talk to you calmly
Appreciate the love and sacrifices that you made for them
That allowed him to be a man and she, a woman
Who could care for their lessened and needy father

1/08

I keep thinking I did the wrong thing when I took Dad home from the nursing home…if only we had the money he could have stayed. But, a sad year later as I look at the notes I took when he was there, I think maybe it wasn't such a bad idea after all. He was so happy to be in my home with sweet, young Monica and the OT he fell in love with twice a week. He sat then at the kitchen table watching me cook and telling me about Aunt Lena until he wandered all through the house at night on his own.

Use every bit of money I have to keep me in my home safely. I have earned that money over a lifetime of hard work and sacrifice. Pay it to a well vetted loving individual who will treat me like family. This person will be hard to find, but if you do due diligence, they are out there. Even though I am taken care of by a special person, call me several times a week and pop in when you can.

Make sure they know who I am before they start getting to know me. Give them all my pictures so we can talk about them. For instance, tell them I must have music, flowers, and books. Tell them your dad loves fishing shows, games on the phone, polenta, or actually anything with red sauce. Maybe drop off your delicious sauce once in a while.

Bring your family to see us as often as you can. If your children are old enough, have them come and spend time with us. This won't be easy but, they will figure it out. And they will be better people for it.

I know it might seem better to put us in a fancy expensive place, and you will use your judgment, but I think we might be happier in our own home with competent people whose job it is to only take care of us.

Of course, the little house on the Coolidge will need some modifications if we stay here, as will most homes. Maybe add a walk-in shower and a toilet right off the kitchen. Dividing up the family room to become a bedroom could work as well.

THINK NOW

Think now about what it means to be independent
Revel in your everyday ability to do as you please
Go where you want
Buy what you want
Say what you want
Do what you want
Be happy you can get up out of bed and go to work
Every day
Because you can
I can't drive or hear others who might still call me
I am isolated from so much of what I used to know
Alone, impotent
This could make me grouchy, pensive, distant, and weird
You can't fix these moods for me really
They have nothing to do with you
Hug me
Know that whatever you do for me will run deep and soothe my soul even if I don't express my gratitude
You can be proud that you were able to love this deeply without much obvious return

7/09

> Put my death notice in the New York Times
> Even if it costs a lot
> For I have had many lives
> That you may not know much about
> Other lonely elders may be looking at the obituaries
> To find and remember an old coworker
> Friend, acquaintance
> Maybe they can travel to say good bye, offer condolences
> Spend some time reminiscing
> Snatching up memories
> And find a moment to be who they once were

If I say at a party "I would love some of that pasta over there!" Do not think you are showing me how much you love me by telling me I am not supposed to have that. Don't say "Have a piece of chicken instead."

Of course, try to see to it that I eat healthily, take my pills, and get out of the house if I can. But, if I say no to the walk because everything hurts, or if I really want that spaghetti, it's okay for you to forget the healthy regimen. I forgive you and I thank you too. When my Dad lived with us, there was a table designated for the sweet treats he loved – Mallomars, Entenmann's cakes, etc. He adored thick shakes!

Again, Let me smoke. There is nothing more fun than to watch an old person light up. I wish I had sat in the garden at the assisted living home with my dad and puffed away together. He would say how much he wanted one and I would laugh. If I knew then what I know now, I would have given him a pack of Kents, a carton. I used to buy them for him at the candy store on the Avenue. He would have one hanging out of his mouth all night long as he worked at the editor's desk at CBS News.

4/22

Yellowed days

Signals to warn

Upcoming reds

When the warnings

Won't help

But just be marks on a calendar

Yes! Again! By all means REVEL in your youth!

Thank God for each day of unencumbered living

Unlimited

Healthy days, salad days

Productive, busy days

Work, walk, laugh days

Baseball, soccer, lacrosse, dance drive days

Can't catch your breath days

Organizing, cleaning, planning your life days

Striving days

The days of your youth are precious

Be healthy, eat right

Exercise

Get an annual physical

Take time for yourself

Be positive

Find a way to de-stress

Maybe your old age will be kind

Maybe it won't

> But you will have tried to make it so
> Most people figure this out
> When they are looking back at the busy times
> And wishing they had taken more care

I do not remember giving pain relievers to my Dad…he had many prescribed pills to take at all hours of the day, but I don't think I gave him anything for pain. I am eleven years younger than he was and I take Tylenol, use Arnica, take hot showers, use heating pads and use ice packs on a regular basis. I guess he did not complain about specific pain for me to think about how I could have helped him to relieve it.

HAIR 4/22

"Gimme a head with hair

Long beautiful hair

Shining, gleaming

Streaming, flaxen, waxen"

HAIR, THE MUSICAL

A symbol of my youth

All youth

The young rebels of the 60s

Amazing, to think of it now

As a statement of revolt

When so many young people today

Shave it off

Or clip it too short, shave off the sides

Long before it is gone

Crop the top

The Beatles with their silly bowl cuts

Were chastened by the elders

Caused a wave in the ocean of post war status quo

"Clean cut" notion ascribed to no more

Of course it wasn't just the hair

Though history showed

Samson's demise without it

On the heads of protestors and rock n roll

Look around at the children of the 60's

Who flaunt their grey tresses or hide their pates under berets or colorful African tams
On stage and off
Hair still representative of who we were
Who we are
"Wow, he looks great" uttered about the lucky guy with hair at 75
Really does not look his age
So when I think of my beautiful mother who took to visiting her beloved Cindy at the neighborhood beauty parlor
Despite the cost
To maintain the red and bouffant of her vibrant youth
The "Red" that my young father lovingly called his high school sweetheart
The "Red" he drew into so many hearts on love letters from the war and handmade cards sent for every occasion
She would often ask me midweek, to tease closed the tiny bald spot at the back of her head
I wish I had better understood
The importance of that small act
One tiny thing
My mother who asked for nothing asked for
And, I, the child of the 60's, begrudgingly complied
As if it were a big favor

Little did I envision myself fast-forward
Peeking into a rear mirror
To see a much bigger bald spot
That requires creative combing, extra time before
I go out
In thankfully, a beret in winter
Shots in my scalp, possible hair extensions,
Jada Pinkett Smith hairdo, prenatal vitamins,
Biotin, Rogaine for Men
Another painful awareness of cycles
Pay attention to elders
As best we can.
My crowning glory, my "lion-hair" of old
Chipping away
If possible, keep my bald spot disguised
Even as you cope with your own.

RUBY RED

Oh, how we laughed
When Auntie called my Dad, crying
That her lips were gone!
Such drama!
Beautiful Auntie says her lips are gone! And I look in the mirror thirty years later and smile a thin-lipped smile.

Ruby red lips
The boys who came to dance at my feet while I sang on the stage
Faces upturned
Lulled by my love songs
Noted forty years later how my ruby red lips lured them
Now I see those lips in the magnified makeup mirror
After almost three years of having to hide them behind Covid masks
The toned down shade of lipstick bleeding up and down into the laugh and smoker's lines
Those once ruby lips much thinner but wrapped around a smile acknowledging my joy at just being here to gaze at them,

CHIPPING AWAY

It's become a joke that we all struggle opening the half and half container
Even Larry David did an episode on the challenge of opening just about any item that's seemingly enclosed for eternity in hard plastic
Limited motion affects all of the things I took for granted
Travel, trips to the city, visits to soccer and baseball games
The world is shrinking
I'm not ready
More to do, more to see!
Forget France
Can't go down a short staircase to do the wash
If I manage that, I can't lift the basket of folded clothes to go back up the stairs
Full of "Can'ts"
A struggle to embrace the gift that each day offers
Constant fight to keep a smile
"Ya gotta laugh" circulating through our peers
"What's your blood pressure doing?"
"Did you get the back, knee, shoulder, hip, ankle shots?"
"What were his inflammation numbers?"
"Have to go, we're doing infusions"

"We're nebulizing"
"When did I take Tylenol last?"
"Did I lose the thermometer again?"
Want to go to a nearby park
Take her to a concert
Run in the wind
Maybe just walk with ease

'TIL SHE CAN'T

There will be a time when I can't do many things
Even simple things
Never mind,
Make a dinner, or set a table
My mom, after a stroke from which she was "recovering", made her mother's crumb cake on the 95 degree day of my husband's birthday because it was his favorite
Died that night, leaving behind a luscious crumb cake as a legacy to her independence

WHILE WE CAN

The list gets shorter every day
Soda bottles
Water bottles
Laundry detergent
Spray cans of this and that
Luckily, the evil COVID days gave way to
Instacart for many of us
Amazon – a lifesaver

You will feel torn between giving proper attention and time to your parent and to your family. Feel safe in the knowledge that you are doing the right thing by seeing to it that your parent is in good hands. Your family will learn about loyalty, sacrifice, and love. They will forgive you for whatever time spent apart from them. Do not fret. As your wise grandfather always said, "This too will pass." You will get back to giving your full attention to your beautiful family soon enough and you will be happy.

A dear friend, who is my age, reflected on her experience taking care of two sets of parents at once. She distilled her advice into one direct statement. Start your journey knowing the fact that YOU CANNOT DO IT ALL. Period. This is a piece of advice that most experienced care givers will give you. It is when you lose sight of this that you can become resentful. She also said that even if you are doing your best, you are often, "damned if you do and damned if you don't." She recounted one of the many times she had experienced this. Her beloved father was at Sloan and dying of cancer. When she arrived to visit him, he was standing out in front of the hospital, with his IV, smoking a cigarette he had bummed from a passerby. Of course, she was taken aback but she did not admonish her dad or tell him to put it out. She reasoned that he should enjoy the time he had left. She later quietly hired an attendant to stay with her dad and make sure he did not go out again. When her brother came to visit that night, her father told him, "I guess I really am a goner. Your sister let me smoke!"

I felt it was very important to speak with other people who experienced taking care of a parent because, despite similarities, every situation is as unique as the folks who are living it. Daughter to mother, son to mother, daughter to father, son to father…each relationship has its own design. There are in-laws and other family too who could be part of that design. There are also children who find themselves caring for a father and a mother at the same time, as well as in-laws who need their help.

Here are but a few suggestions from adult "children" who shared ideas about how to successfully support a parent. Of course, which of these suggestions you choose will depend on "reading the room" as mentioned in number one below.

1. "Read the room": stay very cognizant of what the parent seems to want or need. This will shift from time to time and is hard to decipher if you are not paying close attention. Try to stay realistic even though it is very easy to engage in wishful thinking.
2. Provide projects that you can do together…have all materials and do together e.g. Birdhouse, paint by number, make greeting cards, garden, take notes as parent tells you stories, record conversations. If possible, have your parent help you do simple repairs around the house.

3. Do activities together like looking through pictures, discussing current events. My Dad and I did this all of our lives.
4. Take the parent to an art class or for a pedicure.
5. Take your parent for car rides.
6. Go to stores if the parent is able.
7. Just sit and talk about artifacts that are in the parent's home.
8. Talk about the work that the parent did in his or her life.
9. Talk about what is happening in your life – work, kids, trips, etc.
10. Watch informative or nature TV shows.
11. Listen to the music your parent loves the most. Your Dad loves 50's music!
12. Talk with your parent, remembering he/she is a wise adult. Do not think or act otherwise, despite what you see. But know that "talking" may be a one way street.
13. Expect your parent to do what he or she is able to do. Do not "do for" them if possible. They need to feel capable and as independent as possible.
14. Cook or bake with them.
15. My neighbor read to his wife every day.

16. Go out for lunch or dinner.
17. Just sit together in the sun.
18. My sister-in-law and her husband every year dug and planted a garden for her mom, who loved gardening. When her mom became unable to bend over to pick the fruits and vegetables, they planted a tall container garden that she was able to water, care for, and gather its ripened rewards.
19. Make the home safe by considering the following:

- ✓ If possible, arrange for all of the living space to be on one floor
- ✓ Put the mailbox right outside the door or install a mail slot
- ✓ Organize the pills and write down schedule for taking them
- ✓ Remove all runners and scatter rugs and replace with non-slip mats
- ✓ Move the washer and dryer upstairs
- ✓ Provide written reminders, if necessary, to not go on stairs
- ✓ Put a nightlight in bathroom and bedroom
- ✓ Determine if it is safe to use the stove
- ✓ Put a rubber mat and safety bar in the bathtub

- ✓ Make sure the seating (couch, easy chair) is high enough to get up from without struggling
- ✓ Have a way for the parent to call in an emergency
- ✓ Install a high toilet
- ✓ Install a stair lift if necessary
- ✓ The Internet is a valuable resource. AARP has online articles and tips for how to make a home safe for the elderly.
- ✓ There are many books about caretaking. A friend recommended what she called the "Bible" of caretaker books called, <u>How to Care for Aging Parents</u>, by Virginia Morris.

These suggestions obviously require your time. Make the time to dedicate to your parent. You have to take care of your parent. It is an obligation. "Taking care" can look differently to different people, but the child has to assume this responsibility and play this part in the life scheme of things. Who else will do so? If you were loved and cared for when you were growing up, it is your turn to do the same. Remembering how precious this time can be could help you to embrace this responsibility. Thinking about the things written in this book could help you to be more prepared to manage the caretaking. These strategies could help you to stay the course when you do get overwhelmed. Of course, it is easier when you have a mate, children, and/or siblings who can help figure out the roadmap with you and contribute to easing that load.

Also, if you have two aging parents, be vigilant about knowing when the stronger of the two needs your help. There is a natural division of labor in a long-standing marriage. It is hard just to navigate every day when you are older and have health issues. When you have to take care of yourself and in addition have to care for a less able spouse and do all the chores he or she usually handles, it is very challenging. Figure out ways to ease the burden your "well" parent is carrying.

Some ways I have seen my nieces do this are:

- Visit often
- Regularly, take the "pulse" of the situation concerning both parents
- Do the footwork for arranging for professional support; hire help to come into the home for showers, PT, wound care
- Make the calls for the doctors' appointments
- Make the calls to rectify a problem like the newspaper not coming when it should
- Help plan and arrange for organizing the home so it is easier to navigate
- Take the parent out to hear live music
- Teach the well parent to food shop on line
- Hire helpers to clean and do chores around the house
- Bring cooked food for the freezer

- Cook dinner when you visit.
- Help with the bills
- Make sure someone can take the heavy garbage pail out to the curb
- Have your children visit and/or do Facetime as often as possible
- Help determine when the well parent is no longer able to care for the needy parent

There are obviously many more ways to help that each family can and does figure out. In every situation, the key is AWARENESS. Don't assume that because your parents are in their home and getting through each day that they do not need your help. Even if you are not being asked to help, go there and see what you can do for them.

Positive self- talk is important at every age. In your everyday life, whether you are caring for someone or not, one- liners you might lean on are:

- <u>"You can lead a horse to water, but you can't make her drink."</u>
  You might spend time planning an activity or a way to spend time with your parent on a given day. Be aware that he or she might not feel well enough that day to engage. Don't be disappointed. Hopefully, you can figure out when a bit of coaxing might make it happen or letting it lie would be the better choice. Maybe have a backup way to spend the time. You will probably find

that predictable interactions could work best because there is less disruption in routine or it is an activity you have done before and you know your parent really enjoys it. Tried and true usually works.

- "Suspend logic at times."

    Very often you find yourself thinking that you know what is best for your parent. You can state your case and defend it, but ultimately, they may choose to ignore your advice. You have to let it go. Sometimes you will forget that they are grown, mature adults who have lived a life. They have to be able to do what they want to until they are mentally unable to choose for themselves.

- "Find balance between worrying too much and not enough."

    As mentioned before, what they need will often shift. Being as aware as possible of how they are managing will help you to decide what needs to be done. This is a tough one though. Pay attention to nuances. As your parent gets older, he or she will naturally feel very mortal. Do not think that this is morbid. It makes sense actually. Try to monitor their state of mind in this respect. It is also okay to talk with them about their feelings if you think this might help. I wish I had had some existential talks with my deep-thinking father about this when I could sense that his mortality was on his mind. Every morning when I came to his room, I was afraid of what I would find. This is normal. Of course, worrying will not help this situation. If you have done your best, then you can worry less. This is always true, in every life situation.

- <u>"Embrace every new day that you get to have your parent."</u>
  As you can tell from some of the writings in this handbook, it is challenging to remember to do this, just like it is challenging to embrace every day as a gift, in general. When you are a high performing, logical, problem solver, it can be very hard to accept changes that you see in your parent.

- <u>"This too shall pass"</u>
  There will be good days and bad days. If you take one day at a time, you will realize that one crisis or another will pass. Try to be in the moment and especially enjoy the lulls between the crises. All the clichés and one-liners may seem trivial, but I think they help. Positive self-talk is never going to hurt you.

From my sister-in-law

These suggestions are directed mainly toward caregivers of parents with dementia:

- When you think of someone losing their memory, don't forget that it also encompasses their word association. Understanding what a word means is also memory. So, I will ask mom if she has a bucket, but she cannot picture what that is. Nothing comes into her brain. When she's trying to tell me something, she will describe everything surrounding that word in the hope that I will figure out what she is trying to say.

- Never assume that they understand what you are saying. They are masters of covering up their confusion. You will swear that they understood, but 5 minutes later they have no memory of it. Write down everything for them that you want them to remember. It's not that they're ignoring you or not paying attention. It's just that receptive language is incredibly difficult for them.

- Home is their absolute safe place. It's familiar and constant. So if you invite them over to your house, don't take it personally that they want to go home. It's not that they are having a bad time; it's just that home makes sense to them.

- When you are walking with them, be mindful of contrast. If steps and the landing are the same color, they cannot differentiate where one thing ends and the other begins. It leads to falls.

- People with dementia lose their ability to have empathy. It's not that they don't care; it's just that they are unable to feel that anymore. They cannot grasp the enormity of situations, or the big picture of what it all means.

- Dementia patients have hard time "cross-referencing" information. So, for example, my mom knows that winter weather is cold, but doesn't understand why there

are no flowers in the flower box, or boats on the frozen lake.
- Conversation becomes very difficult. Putting words together and grasping what you're saying is a lot of work. Keep it simple and don't take it personally.
- As dementia progresses they will forget all those stories from the past that they used to repeat constantly. Don't badger them to try to remember. You're frightened and want to "will" them to remember, but they won't. It's ok.
- Vision becomes tricky. They will tell you that they can't see things but when you take them for an eye test their eyes have not gotten worse. The truth is that they are seeing what's around them, but their brain is not processing what it's looking at. The messages are not getting there.
- When you talk about someone they don't see all the time, give them a frame of reference. For example, don't just say "Judy", say Rich and Judy. It's a connector for them.

Note: Realize that Alzheimer's will progress. It is a cruel disease and many of the ways in which you have diligently figured out how to interact with your parent will fade away. As I said before, "Remember I Will Die". Watching a loved one die in stages, losing pieces of themselves, is incredibly heartbreaking. Know that if they are physically here, you still have the opportunity to be there for them. You will see them through loving eyes, saddened, yet determined to be there for them no matter what.

- FIND A CAREGIVER SUPPORT GROUP. It helps you understand that you are not alone. Everyone is going through the same thing you are. They help you understand that all the feelings you are having are normal…The good, the bad, and the ugly. They will remind you to take time for yourself. Go on vacation. If you don't take care of yourself, it will be even more challenging to take care of others.

If I Get Dementia

- I want my friends and family to embrace my reality. If I think my deceased spouse is still alive or if I think we are visiting my parents for dinner, let me believe those things. I'll be much happier for it.
- If I am not sure who you are, do not take it personally. My timeline is confusing to me.
- If I can no longer use utensils, do not start feeding me. Instead, switch me to a finger-food diet, and see if I can feed myself.
- I don't want to be treated like a child. Talk to me like the adult I am even if I cannot talk back.
- Sing with me or to me.
- I still want to enjoy the things that I've always enjoyed. Help me find a way to exercise, dance, listen to music, read, and visit with friends.

- Ask me to tell you a story from my past. Try not to ask me questions.
- Make sure I always have my favorite music playing within earshot.
- Brush my hair.
- Do my nails.
- Rubs my arms with lotion.
- Don't feel guilty. You've done your best.

WHAT I LEFT BEHIND

Every day I get older I look carefully
At my cupboards, my dresser drawers, my closets as I go about my business. I wonder what others will think when I am gone.
I remember cleaning out Mom and Dad's condo after she died, questioning why she had this broken trinket or that worn out blouse
Noticing if there were patterns in how she arranged her clothes or her dishes
Her jewelry
Finding hundreds of safety pins everywhere
I remember she always pinned the front opening of her blouse or it would otherwise be slightly open at the button
What else were these safety pins for?
To help a fellow female worker with a uniform mishap perhaps
Couldn't have that with all of the JPMorgan bankers tended to by her snappy Irish waitresses
Offering a safety pin to someone in need on the train or to hold together a diaper
Just one of the treasures to be found in her pocketbook for any emergency
She was in her early 70's and was obviously aware that we would eventually go through her things because she had a wardrobe of little drawers tucked into her walk-in closet

Each drawer held a precious note to a particular person, willing each a small piece of her costume jewelry to remember her by
Treasures all.
I think of my house! Oh no!
My attic, my garage!
My Mom and Dad had the opportunity to pare down their possessions when they sold their house and moved to Florida
Being here for almost 50 years has allowed no such opportunity!
Living with a pack rat has also made it hard to get rid of things
The basement has become a bit more presentable over time
We have parted with some of the debris from our working years
Plenty of boxes and crates of wonderful awards, notes, and books still remain
Smattering of JP's treasured things down there
Hats, video games and systems, VCR tapes, CDs
My sister, four years my senior, has been steadily emptying her basement filled with the leftovers from three children, student gifts, educational materials, abandoned cribs and baby things, so much that a giant garage sale didn't make a dent
Closure.
I do wonder why my husband doesn't wonder what they will think when they see his garage
He's still too busy using its contents and adding to the "treasures" it houses.

THANK YOU MOM

I did not get to officially or properly thank you for the sacrifices, the hard work, the unconditional love, the positive embrace of life every day, the life lessons
You cooked all day in the heat to make his favorite birthday meal
Polenta and your famous crumb cake
Which sat in the freezer for years before I could let it go.

THANK YOU DAD

Because of you I have known "mothering", "sistering", "daughtering", in these times you have been with me.
I stroked your smooth handsome forehead as you left and I whispered thanks for the love and care that your strong hand gliding across a young girl's feverish brow represented
Even Aunt Lena lived through me for you
Remembering the good life as we hobbled through Now

www.ingramcontent.com/pod-product-compliance
Lightning Source LLC
Chambersburg PA
CBHW031535210526
45464CB00003B/1024